DEPARTMENT OF HEALTH

WELFARE OF CHILDREN AND YOUNG PEOPLE IN HOSPITAL

London: HMSO

Preface

Over the last thirty years, we have come to a better understanding of the unique qualities of children – no longer can they be perceived as just miniature adults! This knowledge has further underlined the importance of the continuing care and support that children need to help them achieve their full potential as adults, and of the expert assistance that parents and carers will sometimes require. Those concerned with the health of children have played a major part in this growth in understanding, and this guide distils the efforts and accomplishments of a wide range of people experienced in all aspects of health care: many have contributed directly through the comments and suggestions they have made during its preparation. The guide aims to convey the results of relevant research, writing and teaching, and the deliberations of expert bodies, but above all, to reflect the quality of widely recognised best practice given to children and their families.

Of the milestones that have led to the preparation of the guide, three are particularly important:

- the Platt report on the Welfare of Children in Hospital[1] which in 1959 first gave recognition to the special needs of children and their families and set in train the pioneering work of the National Association for the Welfare of Children in Hospital in winning recognition of the benefits of involving parents and carers in the health care and treatment of their children
- the Court Report (1976)[2] which recognised the need for integration of children's health services in advocating "a child and family centred service in which skilled help is readily available and accessible; which is integrated in as much as it sees the child as a whole and as a continuously developing person"
- establishing a new service framework for the attainment of these objectives, the White Paper "Working for Patients"[3] which proposed that the new role of District Health Authorities should be to "concentrate on ensuring that the health needs of the populations for which they are responsible are met; that there are effective services for the control and prevention of diseases and the promotion of health; that their population has access to a comprehensive range of high quality, value for money services . .".

The implementation of the Government's reforms to the NHS will enable *Districts* to define explicitly in contracts with *provider units* the standards they require for a high quality child health service and to monitor compliance with these standards. This guide, amplified as necessary by the documents to which it refers, is intended to assist *Districts* in identifying the standards they wish to secure and *providers* in achieving these standards in the delivery of services. It draws on previous Departmental guidance circulars and reflects the consensus of current opinion amongst the professions, managers and other agencies concerned with the health care of children. Pre-eminently, we hope it also reflects the needs and interests of parents and children themselves.

Children are particularly vulnerable to the effects of illness and hospitalisation. Only a short spell in hospital may have a long term effect on the child and family. Children should therefore be admitted to hospital as in-patients only if appropriate care cannot be provided daily or in the community. Whether for in-patients or otherwise, hospital care for children should provide an environment which is conducive to the promotion of health and the lessening of stress, with both emotional and clinical needs receiving constant attention. This is best achieved by grouping children and young people together, and giving families support and encouragement to participate in their care. Children should not be admitted to adult wards as they are not only more emotionally vulnerable than adults but also have different needs, requiring alternative equipment, techniques and staff skills.

Hospital care is only one part of the NHS's responsibility for children. This document emphasises the essential links which have to be forged between hospital services and other NHS primary and community services. It also emphasises the paramount importance of maintaining children's bonds with their families and homes. The integration of children's health services as advocated in the Court Report[2] remains Government policy and, in drawing up contracts, we expect *Districts* to give particular attention to the need for children and their families to receive integrated health care. *Providers* will then need to ensure that their management and organisational arrangements facilitate achievement of this objective.

This guide is the first in a series on Health Services for Children. A similar document will be produced on community health services for children.

Use of the Guide

This guide takes account of recent developments in the care and treatment of children, the management of the NHS and the relationship of the Department of Health (including the NHS Management Executive) to health authorities. The main aim is to bring together in a single document relevant good practice guidance on the care of children in hospital in a form appropriate to the new role of district health authorities and their provider units. As the references indicate, the guidance was drawn from reports and publications by NHS staff, academic departments, professional bodies and voluntary organisations.

Much of the guide comprises standards of care derived from tried and tested good practice. This will assist

- *districts* in developing service specifications for children's hospital services
- *districts* and *provider units* in agreeing contracts for these services
- *provider* units in delivering high quality, efficient services.

In addition we expect the guide to inform the monitoring of the quality of services undertaken by both Regional Health Authorities and the NHS Management Executive. But it will be for *Districts* to judge the relevance of this guidance to their local circumstances and, through the contracts they let, to make any adaptations necessary to fit local practice, or constraints caused by the facilities or resources available.

Throughout the guide good practices are introduced by the phrase "District and Provider Units are advised...". In the few specific instances, however, where it is necessary to be more prescriptive – eg because of legal obligations, the requirements of the statutory and professional bodies responsible for clinical standards or key principles of Government policy for the health care of children – "should..." is used. These instances are

- in placing contracts, account to be taken of government policy for the integration of child health care (paragraph 2.5)
- the statutory requirements on obtaining consent to the treatment of a child (paragraph 3.3)
- the requirement under the Children Act for Local Authorities to be informed when a child has spent 3 months in hospital (paragraph 3.18)
- the need for post-natal mothers, who are transferred from a maternity unit to – for example – a neonatal intensive care unit to remain under the supervision of a midwife (paragraph 4.4)
- the policy requirement that parents/carers should not be charged for the use of facilities to remain overnight with their children in hospital (paragraph 4.9)
- the need for hospitals to collaborate with Local Education Authorities to provide education for children in hospital (paragraph 4.14)
- the need for *districts* and *provider* hospitals to collaborate with Social

Services Departments on the identification, assessment and protection of children at risk (paragraph 4.45 – 4.48)

● the requirements of the Education Acts, the Disabled Persons Acts and the Children Act for health authorities to contribute to the assessment of children's health, educational and social care needs (paragraph 5.1)

● the duties, training and experience required of medical staff in the care and treatment of children (paragraph 6.1)

● the need to ensure that the duties of staff like nursery nurses and health care assistants do not extend to those of a registered or enrolled nurse (paragraphs 6.4 and 6.5).

The guide is generally consistent with the Quality Review "Setting Standards for Children in Health Care"[4] and should provide a complementary source of advice for the quality assurance of children's services.

The appendices comprise a list of references and a bibliography.

Contents

1: Introduction

Illness in Children

1.1 We now have far greater knowledge of how children develop both emotionally and physically. With that understanding has come an awareness of the emotional vulnerability of the young child and the effect which early experience can have on later development. This has influenced how we should care for the sick child. A good quality service for children

- **provides for the child as a whole, for his or her complete physical and emotional well being and not simply for the condition for which treatment or care is required**
- **is child and family centred with children, their siblings and their parents or carers experiencing a "seamless web" of care, treatment and support, as they move through the constituent parts of the NHS.**

1.2 Advances in medicine and improved social circumstances have led to dramatic improvements in child health, but have also created new problems. Conditions, for which until quite recently the prognosis was poor, are being successfully treated. But often these children undergo long and intensive periods of treatment and sometimes remain disabled by mental, physical or sensory impairments.

1.3 Illness in children is always distressing. Serious illness, although fortunately relatively uncommon, is particularly distressing, both to the children themselves and their families. It also requires a highly skilled response from specially trained health service staff which takes account of the developmental differences between the physical, psychological, and physiological needs of sick children and adults. The job of the health service is

- **to promote and preserve good health and prevent illness**
- **where illness does occur, to ensure that children are given the best care and attention in a way that mitigates physical and emotional distress.**

1.4 Flexibility is required in defining childhood. It is generally accepted that children have distinctive health needs until school leaving age (up to age 19) and that adolescents deserve particular attention. In some instances - eg chronic sickness or disability - the transition to adulthood requires close co-operation between children's departments and other specialities.

2: Contracting for Hospital Services

Cardinal principles

2.1 These basic principles inform all aspects of this guide

- **Children are admitted to hospital only if the care they require cannot be as well provided at home, in a day clinic or on a day basis in hospital**
- **Children requiring admission to hospital are provided with a high standard of medical, nursing and therapeutic care to facilitate a speedy recovery and minimise complications and mortality**
- **Families with children have easy access to hospital facilities for children without needing to travel significantly further than to other similar amenities**
- **Children are discharged from hospital as soon as socially and clinically appropriate and full support provided for subsequent home or day care**
- **Good child health care is shared with parents/carers and they are closely involved in the care of their children at all times unless, exceptionally, this is not in the best interests of the child. Accommodation is provided for them to remain with their children overnight**
- **Accommodation, facilities and staffing are appropriate to the needs of children and adolescents and separate from those provided for adults. Where possible separate accommodation is provided for adolescents**
- **Like all other patients, children have a right for their privacy to be respected and to be treated with tact and understanding. They have an equal right to information appropriate to their age, understanding and specific circumstances.**

The Purchaser and Provider Roles

2.2 *District Health Authorities* are responsible for contracting for hospital services for children from NHS Trusts, Directly Managed Units, or private or voluntary hospitals. They will need to contract for a volume and quality of clinical services and make the collaborative arrangements between the hospital services and community and primary care services necessary for delivery of an integrated service. *Districts* are also responsible for **monitoring** the quality of services for which they contract and, with *provider units*, ensuring that there is a clinical audit of these services. DH circular HC (91) 2[5] contains advice on medical audit of hospital and community health services.

2.3 The means by which the required standard of service is secured is a matter for the *District* and the *provider hospital* to agree. In many cases it may be sufficient to draw contractual specifications from the guidance in this document and/or other documents filling a complementary role such as the NAWCH Charter[6] and the NAWCH Quality Review[4]. In some cases - eg the provision of accommodation for parents - *Districts* are advised to make **explicit reference** to the facilities to be provided. The DHA Project Paper "Starting Specifications"[3] summarises lessons learned by Districts and Regions as they prepared specifications for the 1991/92 contracts. It included reference to interim reports from three districts who were using children's services in their contribution to the project. The final versions of these reports, which should be available during 1991, will provide useful guidance in contracting for children's services.

2.4 Some of the issues dealt with in this guidance are relevant to purchasing *Districts*, some to *provider hospitals*. Most will, however, be of interest to both.

Contracting for an integrated pattern of child health care

2.5 In identifying need, planning provision and placing contracts for children's services in hospital, *Districts* and *provider hospitals* should take account of government policy and the general consensus of opinion in favour of an **integrated pattern of care**. Integration means that

- the full range of health services for children - from primary care through health promotion and surveillance to the care of children with special needs and disabilities and the treatment of serious illness - are provided in a **comprehensive and properly co-ordinated manner**
- there is **continuity of care** with children and their parents referred easily and with the minimum of delay to the services they need
- professionals in different parts of the NHS work together with those in other statutory and voluntary agencies to establish effective lines of communication **and constructive** working relationships.

2.6 The main components of this service are

- **a primary care service** for children and their families
- **a comprehensive children's department** incorporating facilities for in-patients, day care, out-patients, treatment of accidents and emergencies and neonatal care
- access to (tertiary) **regional and supra-regional specialities**
- **a community child health service** for pre-school and school-aged children (with close well defined working arrangements with primary care and local authority services)
- **a child development centre** for the assessment and monitoring of children with chronic illness and disability
- **a health promotion** programme relevant to the needs of children and their families.

2.7 In contracting for these services *Districts* will need to assess the local health needs of children and to decide how to secure the integrated provision of services to meet those needs through its management and contractual arrangements. **Continuity, close liaison and the easy flow of appropriate information** between DHAs, FHSAs, hospitals, community health units, GPs, social services departments, education departments and voluntary agencies are essential.

Identifying Need

2.8 In assessing the **volume of hospital services** which they need to purchase for children, *Districts* in consultation with Family Health Service Authorities, Local Authority Social Service Departments and Local Education Authorities are advised to take account of

- **demographic** trends in the child population
- **epidemiological** information on child morbidity
- epidemiological information on **economic, social and psychological**

factors bearing on child health

- any indicators of **unmet need** in respect of acute or chronic illness among the resident child population, eg incidence of children identified as having special educational needs who might have benefited from earlier clinical interventions
- information from research and other sources on the **efficacy of alternative treatments** and the **effectiveness of alternative forms of provision** - the Overview of Research on the Care of Children in Hospital published by the University of Warwick[7] will be helpful here
- the availability of resources.

2.9 *Districts* are then advised to consider, with *providers and GPs*, the developments in the delivery of child health care which have resulted from recognition of the benefits of family centred care - in particular the emphasis on **reducing overnight hospital admissions for children** to a minimum. In striking a balance between hospital and community care account will need to be taken of the extra burden placed on parents and carers by day treatments, **the care of chronically sick children at home and patterns of repeated hospital admission.** Policies and practice on the relationship between **hospital and community** child health services are key issues including

- the use to be made of **paediatric day care** and out-patient facilities
- the services to be provided outside the DGH, eg at specialist clinics to which GPs can refer children for secondary care
- the contribution of **paediatric community nurses** in providing support to families at home, in liaison with GPs and hospitals
- levels of **primary health care services**
- the contribution made by **health visitors and school nurses.**

2.10 Once the contribution of these different elements of the child health service has been agreed, *Districts* will be able to translate their assessment of need into a contractual requirement for hospital care - provided locally, regionally or supra-regionally. This requirement will need to be **regularly reviewed** as better information on the assessment of need becomes available and practices in the delivery of services continue to develop.

2.11 *Districts* will also be responsible for monitoring compliance with their contracts. They are advised to ensure that their information systems distinguish children and young people from other patients in order that the quality and outcome of their care and treatment can be evaluated against the relevant contractual conditions.

3: The Delivery of Hospital Services

The Comprehensive Children's Department

3.1 The desirability of caring for all children within a **Children's Department**, or children's hospital, is well recognised. Grouping children and young people together - preferably with others of their own age group - facilitates the provision of high quality, cost effective care. It enables

- **a children's physician or surgeon** to participate in the general management and professional oversight of the Department (although responsibility for an individual child's medical care may rest with consultants in specialities other than paediatrics)
- children to receive **specialist nursing services**, managed and supervised by, and professionally accountable to, a senior nurse with the **RSCN** qualification (or one who has completed the child branch of Project 2000)
- the **special welfare needs** of children to be more easily met
- **parents/carers and professionals** to share in the care of the child
- **unrestricted** parental involvement during the child's stay in hospital
- an appropriate **child centred routine** in respect of sleeping and feeding patterns
- the provision of **education**
- provision of facilities for **play**
- the environment to be **furnished and equipped** to meet the needs of children.

3.2 *Districts and provider hospitals* are advised to consider the extent to which the children's department can be located on **one site** within the curtilage of the district general hospital. Where, exceptionally it is necessary to accommodate children outside the children's department - eg it may be more appropriate to provide **psychiatric** care for some disturbed children in a small, community-based Child and Family Therapy Unit - discrete facilities offer the most satisfactory solution, managed, as far as is practicable, to the standards set in this document.

Consent to treatment

3.3 *Districts* and *provider hospitals* should ensure that good practices are followed on seeking **consent to the treatment of children**. A guide to consent for examination and treatment published by the NHS Management Executive in August 1990[8] will be of assistance here. The guide indicates that

- the consent of the child and the parent or guardian should be obtained to treat children **under age 16** save in an emergency where there is no time to obtain consent
- normally a child who is seen alone should be encouraged to inform his or her parents except where **it is not in the child's interests to do so**
- there are circumstances where if, in the opinion of a doctor, a child below this age has achieved sufficient understanding of what is proposed, the child **may consent** (or refuse to consent) to a doctor or health professional making an examination and giving treatment (a full note should be made of

the factors taken into account by the doctor in making the assessment of the child's capacity to give consent).

3.4 The rights of children to give consent to treatment were reinforced by a judgement in the House of Lords in 1985 (the Gillick case) which stated that

● "the parental right to determine whether or not their minor child below the age of 16 years will have medical treatment terminates if and when the child achieves a sufficient understanding and intelligence to enable him or her to fully understand what is proposed".

It follows that young people should be kept as fully informed as possible about their condition and treatment to enable them to exercise their rights. Even where younger children do not have the required understanding they should be provided with as much information as possible and their wishes ascertained and taken into account.

3.5 It is essential to establish who is legally responsible for decisions affecting the child and it may be necessary to request copies of any statutory orders. For example, where children are being **looked after** by Local Authority Social Services Departments parental responsibility may be shared or day to day responsibility delegated to a carer (e.g. a foster parent). In certain circumstances **access by a parent may be denied** by a court order. *Provider hospitals* should be alert to these situations in establishing where **primary parental responsibility** lies and who has the right to make decisions on consent to treatment.

3.6 Paragraphs 12 and 13 of the guide[8] give advice on when consent to urgent or life saving treatment for children **is refused by parents/carers** (or by children themselves when judged to be competent).

3.7 The same principles should be followed where consent is sought to the participation of children in medical research. The Royal College of Physician's report "Research Involving Patients"[9] provides relevant guidance.

Accident and Emergency Services

3.8 One third of all patients seen in accident and emergency departments are children and appropriate provision is necessary to meet the needs of children and their families. There are a **range of special provisions** which have become widely accepted as necessary for the successful treatment of children in A&E departments. Often they have been developed in A&E departments in hospitals catering solely for children, but most *districts* will need to purchase at least some of their children's services from units catering for both adults and children. In setting service specifications from *providers, districts* will need to take into account the types of hospital from which they wish to purchase services, the need for families within a well-populated community to have easy access to a children's A&E department and the desirability of the department being located on the same site as the children's hospital. The Royal College of Nursing report "Nursing Children in the Accident and Emergency Department"[10] provides a useful guide to good practice.

3.9 *Districts* and *provider hospitals* are advised to consider the following standards

- provision of **appliances and equipment appropriate for the treatment of children** - eg child size resuscitation equipment
- separate waiting space, play facilities and examination, treatment and recovery rooms furnished and equipped to meet children's needs in safe conditions
- access for parents and carers to **examination, x-ray and anaesthetic rooms** in order that they may be involved in these procedures - eg by calming and comforting their child
- effective procedures to **prioritise waiting children** and ensure they are seen promptly
- the availability, at all times, of medical and nursing staff **trained and experienced in the care and treatment of children**
- the **training of non-paediatric staff** in communicating with children, the sympathetic handling of children and their families and the use of drugs and equipment for the treatment of children
- policies which ensure that **health promotion** opportunities offered by the attendance of children and their families at A&E departments are fully exploited
- a defined policy on the handling of **children in need of protection** and/or suspected of having suffered abuse (see paragraphs 4.45 – 4.48)
- procedures and facilities for counselling, comfort and support of parents in the event of the **sudden death** of a child (see paragraph 4.2)
- effective procedures for communicating with GPs, health visitors, community health staff and social workers: HN(84) 25/LASS(84)5[11] contains guidance on the need for the early involvement of the child psychiatric team where children or adolescents are suspected of having **harmed themselves deliberately**
- procedures for **discharge** which ensure that parents are given all necessary information about the further care of their child and that the GP is notified promptly of the arrangements and any continuing treatment needs (see paragraphs 3.19-3.22)
- procedures for **in-patient admission** which ensure that children are referred without delay to a children's ward with all relevant information (including leaflets on admission procedures etc) provided to the parents (see paragraphs 3.13-3.18) - these procedures should cover instances where the transfer/transport of the child to hospital is necessary.

Out-patients

3.10 Most children are seen first in out-patients departments and this **first impression of the hospital environment can be a strong influence** on the response of these children and their families to hospital care. Wherever possible, separate out-patients facilities for children should be provided. If planning permits, siting the children's OPD in close **proximity to the children's department enables the most effective use** to be made of staff and facilitates the development of a co-ordinated service.

3.11 In setting specifications for out-patient services, *Districts* will need to take account of the siting of these facilities in provider hospitals. If a separate OPD cannot be provided, *Districts* are advised to specify that either a **discrete area** within the adult department is designated for children with appropriate staffing and equipment or certain times are designated for the exclusive attendance of children. Similar provision for children is required in the x-ray department waiting area.

3.12 Whatever the siting arrangements, *Districts* and *provider hospitals* are advised of the following good practices in the delivery of children's out-patient services

- **individual appointments** made to ensure lengthy waiting times are avoided
- the presence of a **RSCN** (or a nurse who has completed the children's branch of Project 2000) at all times
- provision of **child-sized furniture**, low toilet seats and wash-hand basins, and toys and children's books to create a welcoming environment
- facilities for **weighing and measuring children** - in privacy where it is necessary to obtain an accurate unclothed weight
- facilities including a separate interview room for children or adolescents who require **psychiatric therapy** to be seen with their families
- recognition of the particular needs of frail children and children (or **parents/carers) with disabilities** including the provision of ramps and automatic doors and staff with experience of physical and sensory impairment to give appropriate advice to OPD staff
- a designated and suitably equipped **play area**, supervised by a play specialist
- facilities for parents/carers accompanying children including an area for mothers to **breast feed** their babies and change infants and toddlers
- the availability of **refreshments and a telephone** from which external calls may be made (these facilities may be particularly appreciated by families who have travelled a long distance)
- **good access** at all doors for wheelchairs and double pushchairs
- **a safe area** in which prams and push chairs can be parked
- **availability of information** for children and parents attending the OPD including the provision of signs and literature in ethnic community languages where this is appropriate
- the arrangement of out patient sessions in **outreach clinics or peripheral hospitals** which reduce travelling by children and their families.

Admission to hospital

3.13 In planning provision and placing contracts *Districts* and *provider hospitals* are advised to ensure that

- children are usually treated in their **own homes** by the primary care services, with help as necessary from elsewhere in the NHS - eg community paediatric nurses - and other agencies such as social services and education departments
- if hospital treatment is necessary, children should be seen wherever possible as **out-patients or day patients** rather than being admitted to hospital
- in certain circumstances, such as for counselling or familiarisation prior to admission, investigation, or follow-up after discharge, **children may attend the ward without formal admission** as a day case or in-patient.

3.14 To meet these principles, contractual specifications, or the understandings which underpin them, will need to provide for **support from hospitals** to enable as many children as possible to be treated in their homes for as long as clinically appropriate. In some cases children are still admitted to hospital because simple therapeutic materials are not readily available for use at home. In such cases the *District* and the *provider hospital* are advised to look at ways in which **facilities, equipment and/or materials could be loaned** under the supervision of general practitioners or community health staff. Where they exist paediatric community nursing services can make a very helpful contribution to the support of families caring for sick children at home.

3.15 Where admission is essential, the following good practices have been widely adopted for planned admissions

- **procedures which ensure that the child and parents/carers are informed in age-appropriate manner** of the name of the consultant, the reason for the admission, its expected duration, the nature of the treatment with its prognosis and significant side effects
- arrangements for families **to visit the ward** prior to admission - eg at an out-patient visit - to familiarise themselves with the environment and procedures
- procedures which ensure that at this visit or on some other suitable occasion parents/carers are **encouraged to remain with their child** throughout the admission and given information about accommodation and facilities provided for them
- the issue of guidance leaflets to parents, in **ethnic community languages** where appropriate, which include information on what children may/need to bring with them (clothes, toys etc), suggestions as to how parents can reassure their children about attending hospital, and the address of the Community Health Council
- the issue to children of **guidance material related to their age.**

3.16 These procedures should not overlook the possibility that the parents/carers may be disabled and would be assisted by

- information on **physical access** to all parts of the hospital
- **alternative forms of admission information** – tape for people with visual impairments, sign language interpreter for the deaf
- **sensitivity** in ensuring that disabled parents are as involved in the hospital treatment of their children as other parents and carers.

3.17 In the event of an **emergency**, admission procedures should exist for providing families with admission guidance as soon as practicable.

3.18 The 1989 Children Act contains a requirement that local authorities be informed when a child has spent or is likely to spend 3 months in a NHS or private health establishment. *Districts* **should ensure** arrangements exist in *provider hospitals* for these notifications.

Discharge from hospital

3.19 Children are especially **vulnerable** to any shortcomings in hospital discharge arrangements – particularly those who are at risk of abuse, have long term disabilities or whose parents seem unable or unwilling to care for them. Community paediatric nursing services can play a particularly useful part in supporting families care for their children on discharge from hospital

3.20 Health Circular HC(89) 5[12] required health authorities to ensure that wards and departments maintain **up to date discharge procedures** of which all staff with relevant interests are made aware. *Districts* are advised to ensure that the units from which they purchase children's services have procedures which:

- **define the responsibilities** of all those involved - the different hospital staff groups, ambulance staff, members of the primary care team, local authority staff and any voluntary bodies concerned
- include arrangements for **timely communication** between these staff
- require the allocation - to a named member of staff - of responsibility for **ensuring that these procedures have been completed** before a patient is discharged.

3.21 The circular goes on to emphasise the need for planning of discharges and lists the features of a good quality discharge procedure which, in terms of hospital care for children, involve

- an opportunity for hospital staff to discuss with the child's family, prior to admission if possible, the likely outcome and length of stay and the kind of **support the family might require after discharge**
- early assessment of the **suitability of the home circumstances** for the child's discharge, the type of support the family will require and any adaptations or equipment necessary for the child to be cared for at home
- liaison with the Social Services Department about families who may require **social support** or, if it appears that the child may not be able to return to the family home (eg a child **at risk of abuse**), about alternative care and accommodation arrangements
- discussion of arrangements for discharge with the family or other carers **before** they are finalised
- timely notification to **the GP**, with discussion where necessary, of the date of the child's discharge, the diagnosis, the appropriate medication and the arrangement of any continuing care
- timely notification to the child's health visitor by the **liaison health visitor**
- liaison between hospital and **community therapists** – eg physiotherapists – assisting in the care and treatment of children with chronic illnesses such as cerebral palsy and cystic fibrosis
- liaison with the community child health team on continuity of support and **integration into nursery, playgroup or school** as appropriate
- arrangement of **transport for** the child and, if necessary, members of the family
- provision to the parents/carers of any **necessary equipment, dressings or medicines** with instructions on their use and information on dietary arrangements and all other aspects of their child's care - preferably, oral communications should be reinforced with written instructions
- notification to the parents of arrangements made for any out-patient attendance or other **follow-up treatment** by the hospital (eg ward attendance).

3.22 To ensure that no child's **return home** is delayed unnecessarily arrangements for continuing care in the community should be made early in the planning of discharge. It is good practice, where it is appropriate to their care and treatment, for children to be allowed home at weekends or at other times convenient to the family. It is very important that the **GP is aware** of such arrangements. The family may be eligible for help with travel costs (see paragraph 4.7)

Ward Attenders

3.23 The number of children visiting in-patient paediatric and other departments as "ward attenders" - often for follow-up after an in-patient admission - has increased in recent years. When planned, the practice is appreciated by both hospital staff and children and their families in providing informal continuity of care. It was the subject of a study by Caring for Children in the Health Services - Hidden Children[13] – which suggested that the practice worked most satisfactorily when **there were close links between hospital children's departments and community health services for children.** In contracting for children's services *Districts* and *provider units* are advised to take account of the resource requirements generated by ward attenders and the following recommendations of the CCHS report

- **data** is collected on the child ward attenders and the procedures undergone (introduction of the Körner Hospital Episode System is helpful here)
- the care of the children is **supervised by a Registered Sick Children's Nurse** (or one who has completed the child branch of Project 2000)
- ward attendance by children **is monitored** to check that a good quality service is delivered and that the practice is not being used to compensate for deficiencies in other areas of service such as out-patient and community services for children.

Day patients

3.24 Day care can make a valuable contribution to family centred health care by **reducing the occasions when it is necessary for a child to be admitted overnight in hospital.** It also offers a more efficient use of hospital facilities. But, as in other areas of children's health care, special provision needs to be made for their needs; policies for the care and treatment of adult day cases are not capable of meeting these needs. "Just for the Day" published by the Caring for Children in the Health Services consortium (CCHS)[14] provides a very full account of the issues to be addressed in the management and delivery of day care for children. A study conducted by the NHS Management Executive Value for Money Unit - "Organisation and Costs of Day Surgery"[15] is another useful reference document.

3.25 In recent years an increasing number of investigations and elective surgical operations have been carried out on children as day patients in out-patient departments, in-patient wards and, increasingly, in children's day units integral to the children's department. **The organisation and location of children's day facilities** will be for *provider hospitals* to decide in the light of the specifications agreed with the *Districts* and consultation with GPs. They are advised to consider the following standards

- the treatment programme is planned to cater for the pre-admission, treatment and discharge including all necessary liaison with primary and **community health services** and the arrangement of follow-up consultations
- the child is neither **admitted nor treated alongside adult patients**
- the child is cared for by staff especially designated to children's day care
- medical, nursing and other staff are trained and experienced in the care and treatment of **children** as day cases
- the patient management system is designed for **every child to be discharged within the day** except, rarely, when complications render this impracticable
- the environment is suitably laid out and furnished with **easy access for**

people with disabilities and an area where children can play before and after treatment.

3.26 In meeting these standards, *provider hospitals* are likely to have 4 main options

- creation of a discrete **children's day unit**
- planned and designated use of a **separate area in a children's inpatient ward**
- designation of a **separate area within a day care unit**
- designation of **certain sessions within a day care unit for children's treatments** – eg a "children's day" once a week.

3.27 The main determinants are likely to be the level of demand for day treatments and the availability of suitable accommodation in relation to the operating theatres and children's in-patient facilities. The CCHS[14] study advocates that, wherever practicable, **discrete** units should be established within the children's department but, whatever arrangements are made, *provider hospitals* are advised the following good practices

- provision of suitably furnished and equipped accommodation – e.g. with child-proof fittings - for the attendance of children and their parents/carers, **separate** from both that for adult day care and in-patient children
- a treatment room fitted with **appropriately sized equipment**, if anaesthetics are to be administered it must be fully equipped to operating theatre standards
- the **designation** of management and professional staff responsible for the unit including RSCNs (or nurses who have completed the child branch of project 2000), play specialists and administrative staff capable of carrying out admission and discharge procedures to time
- the **provision of children's in-patient beds** to which children can be admitted with minimum disruption if an overnight stay is necessary.

Neonatal Services

3.28 The care of children starts before and at birth. Well newborn babies are cared for by their mothers, assisted by the midwife under the supervision of a paediatrician. Guidance on neonatal care is contained in the third report of the Maternity Services Advisory Committee[16]. The report emphasises the paramount need in the postnatal period for babies to be cared for alongside their mothers. If a newborn baby is small and/or ill, special and intensive care facilities are required staffed by paediatricians, neonatal nurses and midwives. **Ideally maternity and paediatric departments should be located close together on the same site.** Whatever the siting arrangements, close collaboration is required between management of the two services to ensure that the needs of newborn babies and their families are met with high quality services.

3.29 In setting service specifications *Districts* are advised of the need for policy decisions to be taken on the organisation and delivery of normal, special baby and neonatal intensive care covering

- the designation of **different levels of care** related to the condition and birthweight of the baby
- the facilities required – **number of normal, special and/or neonatal**

intensive care cots

- the location of these facilities including, where appropriate, **access to regional specialist facilities.**

3.30 In agreeing contracts *Districts* and *provider hospitals* are advised of the following standards

- a consultant paediatrician is available **24 hours a day** to supervise the care of newborn babies
- sufficient **specially trained medical, midwifery and nursing staff** are also always available to meet routine and emergency needs of newborn babies including the staffing of any special or intensive care cots
- well established procedures exist for the **identification of babies requiring specialist facilities** and their timely transfer to an appropriately staffed and equipped specialist unit
- encouragement is given to medical and nursing staff to develop their skills in neonatal care through **formal and informal training opportunities**
- facilities are provided in neonatal units for parents/carers to **remain with their babies** and, as far as practicable, they are encouraged to participate in their care
- **support and counselling** is available for families with very ill or small babies and for families and staff in the event of a baby's death (see paragraph 4.42).

The Paediatric Intensive Care Service

3.31 The British Paediatric Association Working Party on Paediatric Intensive Care[17] defines the function of a Paediatric Intensive Care Service, as providing "for the needs of the critically ill child **requiring constant individualised nursing care and immediately available skilled medical help.**"

3.32 Many critically ill children are still admitted to adult intensive care units where the majority of patients are adults. The BPA report[17] recommends that, in these situations, admissions should be notified to staff in the paediatric department and their co-operation sought to ensure that the child is cared for in a suitable environment **separate from adults**.

3.33 Whether the service is to be provided in a discrete children's unit or in a designated area within an adult ICU, *Districts* and *provider hospitals* are advised to agree on the following standards for paediatric intensive care

- the nurse in charge has a **RSCN** qualification (or has completed the child branch of Project 2000) and preferably has attended one of the English National Board courses leading to a recordable qualification in the intensive care nursing of children
- the skill mix and numbers of suitably qualified nurses is appropriate to the **degree of dependency** of the children cared for
- facilities for parents/carers to **remain with their children overnight** are available and, where appropriate, they are encouraged and enabled to be participants in the care of their children
- **play facilities** are available under the supervision of a play specialist for those children able to benefit from them
- there should be **training** opportunities for staff – eg nurses and physiotherapists – to develop their skills in intensive care nursing and, in recognition of the demands made upon them, support services available for them to discuss their experience.

Isolation

3.34 Isolation facilities are required to prevent the spread of certain infectious diseases and to protect children whose **immune systems are suppressed**. *Districts* are advised to consider the need for isolation facilities in their contracts for children's services. The Department has guidance on isolation facilities in hospitals in preparation which will emphasise the need for hospital staff and members of the child's family to follow the procedures laid down by the hospital infection control team.

3.35 *Provider hospitals* are advised to take account of guidance in Hospital Building Note No 23[18] on the use of appropriately equipped **single-bed cubicles** for children who are highly susceptible to infection or suffering from infections which could spread to other children. Accommodation for parents and carers can usually be provided within the cubicle. Experience shows that, with the increasing and welcome trend in managing children with infectious diseases in children's wards, **the ratio of cubicles to open beds may need to be increased.**

3.36 Special efforts are necessary to ensure that children who need to be treated in a degree of isolation are included as far as possible in ward activities and do **not suffer unnecessary discrimination.** Play specialists can make a very useful contribution here.

Specialist Hospital Services for Children

3.37 Although a comprehensive children's department fits well into the concept of local provision at the local NHS Trust or directly managed District General Hospital, provision of highly specialised services will often need to be provided at, and contracted from, **regional or supra-regional centres**. In contracting for these services *Districts* are advised to ensure that

- wherever possible, children are referred to the centre which is nearest to, or most accessible to, their home and family
- **adequate transport arrangements** are made for children (and parents/carers), who may be very sick, including provision for appropriate specialist staff to accompany the children to the specialist centre
- regional and supra-regional services **meet the standards and principles of care in this document** – particularly those regarding the involvement of paediatricians and specialist children's nurses in the care of children wherever they are admitted to hospital
- regional specialists are encouraged to develop **peripatetic clinics in DGHs** so that their expertise can be made available to children nearer their homes.

Examples of such regionally specialised services are:

Regional
Plastic surgery/burns
Neurology/neuro-surgery

Specialist genetic services
Neonatal and paediatric surgery
Paediatric urology and nephrology
Paediatric oncology
Bone marrow transplantation
Cystic fibrosis
Growth and endocrinology
Hepatology
Neonatal intensive care
Regional comprehensive assessment (in
support of district services) in relation to
complex handicap and neurology
Paediatric cardiology and cardiac surgery
Specialist paediatric infectious disease
(including the management of HIV)
Paediatric rheumatology
Paediatric radiology and imaging
Paediatric pathology

Supra-regional
Cranio-facial surgery
Endoprosthetic services for primary bone
tumours
Heart transplantation
Liver transplantation
Neonatal and infant cardiac surgery
Specialised liver services
Spinal injury services

Psychiatric services for the deaf
Retinoblastoma service
Stereotactic radiosurgery

3.38 The Department plans to produce guidance on the health and social care of children and families affected by **HIV and AIDS**. It is important that children with HIV and AIDS are seen first as children and that children's departments have the skills and equipment to nurse immuno-suppressed children (see paragraph 3.34 – 3.36)

4: Meeting Children's Special Needs

Parental Attendance and Involvement

4.1 A cardinal principle of hospital services for children is complete ease of access to the child by his or her parents, and to other members of the family (as well as a mother or father "a parent" could be a grandparent, uncle, aunt, sibling, nanny or close friend of the family). This is not a luxury. It is now generally accepted that the care and comfort of parents for a child is fundamental to the care and treatment of children in hospital. The care provided by a hospital has to centre firmly on the recognition of the **child as a member of a family** – a family whose support during the hospital stay is essential to the child's well being. The presence of members of the family is not only a preventative and therapeutic measure, it also provides for the education of the family in both the clinical condition from which the child is suffering and areas like parentcraft and health promotion. The report Hidden Children[13] showed the amount of nursing time spent in **educating families so that they were confident and competent in taking over care of their child on discharge.**

4.2 *Districts* and *provider hospitals* are advised to agree service specifications which

- recognise that parents and members of the immediate family are not visitors and encourage and assist them to be with their child **at all times** unless the interests of the child preclude this
- enable parents to give continuous **love, care, comfort and support to their child** and, especially, be together with their child at the most stressful times - eg during and after treatment, anaesthesia, investigations and x-rays
- **help parents** themselves to undertake many familiar tasks helpful to the care of their child (eg dressing and undressing) and, where appropriate, learn any clinical procedures which will enable them to care for their child at home after discharge
- provide maximum help and advice to parents to enable them to play a part in the care of their children and **to continue the care** following the child's discharge from hospital
- ensure that, exceptionally, when consideration is given to advising a parent on medical grounds **not to visit** a particular child, the decision is taken by the consultant in charge only after **full consultation** with other professional staff (the reasons for the decisions will need to be recorded in the child's medical records)
- enable parents to comfort their children during the **induction** of anaesthesia and to be present during post-operative recovery (if there are good reasons for a parent not to do so, these should be clearly explained)
- ensure, in those instances where a child is unaccompanied on admission to hospital, that efforts are made **to identify the child's carer** calling upon the assistance of hospital social workers as necessary.

4.3 Contact with the family is especially important with those children who require **longer-stay care** in hospital (for example, very small ill babies in a regional neonatal centre a great distance from the family's home, when there may be other children at home). For children of all ages the difficulties created in maintaining family links may lead to **rejection and abandonment**, especially where there is inadequate communication between hospital staff and parents. Where this is felt to be a risk, the co-operation of the social work staff should be sought. There are a number of voluntary organisations which help families with children suffering from serious or chronic illness - some are even able to provide accommodation for families near regional centres in specialities like paediatric oncology. *Provider hospitals* are advised to collaborate with such organisations and to ensure that the services they offer are appropriately publicised.

4.4 The Maternity Services Advisory Committee (MSAC)[16] in its third report recommends unrestricted access **by parents to their baby.** The report recommends that where babies are transferred to another hospital or to another part of the hospital e.g. the paediatric department, specific arrangements should be made for the parent/carer to stay there. Postnatal mothers who transfer to another hospital to be with their sick baby should be kept under the supervision of a midwife - this can often be arranged by the community midwifery service.

4.5 *Provider hospitals* are advised to give every encouragement to mothers who choose to **breast feed** their baby and provide space where they can do this in a degree of privacy. A breast feeding mother may need to be assisted to provide milk if this is what she wishes. It may mean storing labelled bottles of her expressed breastmilk in a refrigerator to give to the baby while she is absent (The Chief Medical Officer's letter on HIV Infection, Breast Feeding and Human Milk Banking-PL/CMO(89)4[19] advises on the handling of expressed milk).

4.6 *Districts* are advised to consider, with *provider hospitals*, what facilities are required **to enable parents to stay overnight** with their children and ensure they are provided for in contracts. The CCHS report "Parents Staying Overnight with their Children in Hospital"[20] suggested the following needs

- **a variety of accommodation** depending upon the child's needs, eg a folding bed by the child's bed, a bed in the parents room or in a hostel near the hospital
- washing facilities, use of a sitting room, kitchen, toilets and access to a telephone
- in specialist hospitals (distant from the family home) **accommodation for siblings** as well as parents.

Health Building Note No 23 "Hospital Accommodation for Children"[18] gives design guidance on facilities for parents/carers (recent experience suggests that more accommodation for parents to stay overnight is required than is suggested in the building note).

4.7 Escorting and visiting children in hospital may impose an additional **financial strain** on families. *Provider hospitals* are advised to ensure that the hospital travel costs scheme is publicised within the children's department and that a named member of staff is designated to help advise families on the benefits which may be available to them in these circumstances. (Leaflet H11 describes how families in receipt of Income Support or Family Credit, or on low incomes can receive help from the Hospital Travel Costs Scheme[21]).

4.8 Where a family's financial situation is particularly difficult, parents should be aware of any assistance the **hospital social worker can provide**. Some bus operators are offering **concessionary fares** to parents visiting children in hospital on production of passes which are issued by the operator to hospitals. If approached, *provider hospitals* are asked to co-operate by making arrangements for passes to be completed for parents with children in hospital.

4.9 Because parents/carers are essential for the well-being of the child in hospital, **no charge should be made for their accommodation.** The question of whether any charges should be made for other services (eg meals) is one for determination between the *District* and *provider hospital*, but it is suggested that parents/carers, whether or not they stay overnight, should be offered the benefit of any subsidised canteen meals.

The Role of Play

4.10 Two recent publications contain advice and guidance on the provision of play in hospital:

- The Play in Hospital Liaison Committee publication "Quality Management for Children: Play in Hospital"[22]
- The Save The Children Fund publication "Hospital: A Deprived Environment for Children? The Case for Hospital Playschemes"[23]

4.11 They show that **play is essential** to the intellectual, social and emotional development of children. It can also help them resolve stressful situations like admission to hospital where they may have to undergo painful treatment procedures and suffer separation from family and friends. Parents who accompany their children on admission to hospital may find it difficult to devote all their time to one child without the interruptions provided by the daily round of chores. Participation in an organised play scheme may, in such circumstances, be a welcome normalising activity. Research shows that play reduces anxiety, facilitates communication and **speeds recovery and rehabilitation**. Play specialists in hospitals can

- contribute to **clinical judgements** through their observation and communication with children
- help **prepare children** for diagnostic tests, surgery and other invasive procedures
- identify children or members of their families who are distressed or **having difficulty coping**
- organise play to provide **diversional therapy**
- introduce some **normality** into a child's day by relieving boredom through a structured programme of developmental activity.

4.12 *Districts* are advised to ensure that *provider hospitals*

- provide **play facilities** in all areas of the hospital in which children are cared for
- employ hospital **play specialists** to run play schemes
- establish well defined lines of **accountability** for play specialists within the hospital management structure to achieve effective and efficient management

of this activity

- facilitate **close collaboration with other specialist staff** concerned with children's care and rehabilitation - eg physiotherapists.

4.13 *Provider hospitals* are advised to ensure that

- there is **adequate separate accommodation** for play with easy access to all children including those who are bed bound and those with sensory and physical disabilities using wheelchairs and other aids to mobility (Health Building Note 23[18] suggests how this accommodation can be provided)
- there are **toys** and other necessary equipment provided in these areas.

Education

4.14 The importance of providing education for children in hospital is generally recognised; children in hospital need access to education to minimise the impact of the **interruption to their schooling** and to provide stimulation. Play is essential for children of all ages but it is no substitute for education for children of statutory school age (5-16 years). Although hospital schools are not formally required to provide the **National Curriculum** under the Education Reform Act 1988, DES circular 5/89[24] makes it clear that such schools and other educational provision in hospital should aim to meet the requirements of the National Curriculum in respect of short-stay and long-stay patients. The HMI report "Hospital and Home Tuition"[25] and the DES publication "Hospital and Home Education Services"[26] contain guidance and information on good practice in this area.

4.15 Section 56 of the Education Act 1944[27] empowers Local Education Authorities (LEAs) **to provide appropriate education** for all children of statutory school age who would be receiving education but for their stay in hospital and who are fit to benefit from it. Under section 3 of the 1981 Education Act[28] LEAs also have discretionary powers, after consulting the parents, to arrange for children with special educational needs (SEN) to receive education otherwise than in schools. *Provider hospitals* are required to provide for the **accommodation needs of children** receiving education in hospital, but may seek a contribution to the capital and running costs of this accommodation from LEAs (Department of Education and Science (DES) Design Note 38[29] contains guidance on meeting the educational needs of children in hospital).

4.16 The physical punishment of children in maintained schools - including hospital schools - is now illegal. As in all other areas of a hospital, children **should never be punished by smacking, slapping or shaking.**

4.17 *Districts* should ensure that *provider hospitals* collaborate with LEAs to provide and maintain

- **facilities** (including equipment and apparatus) for education of school age children in hospital
- good practice to **modify unacceptable behaviour** in children
- procedures for liaison with LEAs on **notification of the admission of children to hospital** who are likely to remain in hospital long enough and be well enough to benefit from education
- **access to records** for hospital teachers so that they have sufficient data to submit returns for inter-LEA recoupment purposes

- **education for children in special circumstances** such as children admitted to adult wards, children up to 19 years with SEN and children under 5 who have already been identified as having SEN
- the maintenance of **links with the school** in the child's home area to achieve continuity of education.

4.18 Specific guidance on the education of **children and young adults** with **mental handicap** in hospital is contained in DES Circular 5/74 issued under cover of HSC(IS) 37[30].

Children with Special Educational Needs

4.19 Statutory assessment procedures under Section 5 of the Education Act 1981[28] may be required for some children in hospital, eg if the child

- has severe or complex **learning difficulties**
- has a **medical condition** likely to affect future learning ability
- was admitted in connection with **a social condition** (such as social deprivation, whether negligence, neglect or child abuse) which is likely to affect future learning ability
- is receiving treatment likely to affect **future learning ability**
- has been admitted to a child or adolescent **psychiatric ward** (psychiatrists should always take education into account in devising programmes for the care and treatment of mentally ill children).

4.20 In all these circumstances the *provider hospital* should liaise with the DHA-designated Medical Officer, so that he or she can inform the LEA and the LEA can form a judgement as to whether the child can be **assessed or reassessed**. Liaison with the Social Services Department may also be necessary.

4.21 Detailed guidance on the implications for the NHS of the 1981 and 1988 Education Acts is given in joint DES/DH Circular 22/89 issued under cover of HN(89)20[31]. On site teachers can give advice on the care and facilities required by children with a range of Special Educational Needs.

Children with Disabilities

4.22 A child with disabilities who has to be admitted to hospital is **doubly disadvantaged**. *Districts* and *provider hospitals* are advised to ensure facilities, procedures and staff are able to cope with the special needs of children with a physical, intellectual, sensory or communication disability who have to be admitted to a (general) paediatric ward when they are receiving treatment for a condition other than their disability.

4.23 Children with sensory impairments are vulnerable to isolation and the deprivation of information normally assimilated by sight and hearing may add to the stress of being in hospital. The special needs of these children should be taken into account in the training of staff and the arrangement of care programmes. Particular regard should be paid to ensuring that

- staff have a **good knowledge of a range of special educational needs** including those of blind/visually impaired, deaf/hearing impaired, deaf/blind and speech disordered children and develop good contacts with LEA specialist support services to enable effective action to be taken as soon as a child with such needs is admitted to hospital
- there is close liaison with the child's school

- when a child has a communication disability, staff are informed of the child's **preferred mode of communication** and information given to the child in suitable form, eg large print or braille texts, word or picture charts, sign language (appropriate interpreter services will be helpful here)
- children with physical disabilities, along with all other children are helped to maintain their **independence and skills**
- parents/carers are encouraged to bring in special seating/equipment/toys **used by their child** – if these are not available the advice of an occupational therapist should be sought
- the family receive advice on the **financial and emotional burden** caused by frequent admissions of a child to hospital.

4.24 **Respite care** provides essential support to families with children with disabilities. (see paragraph 5.13 – 5.16).

Children from Ethnic, Religious or Cultural Communities

4.25 *Districts* and *provider hospitals* need to be sensitive to the individual needs of children and families from minority groups of different ethnic, religious or cultural composition. The following reports provide guidance on these issues:

- "Action not Words - A Strategy to Improve Health Services for Black and Minority Groups"[32]
- "Health Care in Multiracial Britain"[33] and "Traveller Mothers and Babies"[34]

4.26 Parental culture is derived from family tradition in the way children are fed, clothed and comforted. Hospital routines need to be sufficiently **flexible to adapt to different practices.** The translation of patient/parent information into minority languages and the use of interpreters can help families adjust to the hospital environment, especially if parents are given positive encouragement to express their cultural preferences for the care of their children. *Provider hospitals* may need to make enquiries of the communities on how to provide for these preferences which may relate to

- **diet and feeding**
- **clothing** including night clothing and preparation for medical examinations and other interventions
- **washing and bathing**
- religious beliefs or traditions in respect of healing, medical treatment and **care while dying.**

4.27 Certain **inherited conditions** are especially prevalent among ethnic communities - eg sickle cell disease and thalassaemia. Where diagnosis of such a condition - in trait or disease form - is made, expert screening advice needs to be made available to all family members. It may be appropriate to delay advice on the implications for parenting until the family have been counselled on the significance of the diagnosis for their child.

Arrangements for Adolescents

4.28 The NAWCH publication "Setting Standards for Adolescents in Hospital"[35] contains guidance on the care and treatment of adolescents in hospital.

4.29 The impact of the physiological, social, intellectual and emotional changes which adolescents experience is likely to be intensified by hospital admissions through acute or chronic illness. Adolescents have **distinctive and different**

needs from both child and adult patients.

4.30 As children mature at different rates, **flexibility** is necessary in identifying adolescent patients. Most children will be experiencing some kind of developmental change by the start of the teens which can extend to and sometimes beyond school leaving age. Assessment of the need for hospital care will depend upon District policies and past experience. A British Paediatric Association Working Party on the Needs and Care of Adolescents (1985)[36] concluded that the need for hospital beds was least in the age group 11-15 years with **general and orthopaedic surgery** accounting for 40% of bed needs. Needs rise in the 15 to 19 age group as a result of a higher incidence of **trauma** and **road traffic accidents.**

4.31 *Districts* and *provider hospitals* are advised of the following good practices for the hospital care of adolescents

- the accommodation of adolescent patients in a separate unit from children's and adult wards within children's departments which can provide privacy, **flexibility of regime and independence**
- space for **socialising, hobbies, homework** or just to be alone
- **involvement** of adolescent patients in their treatment - whilst retaining close links with their families, many adolescents value the opportunity to make decisions which affect their life-style and development.

4.32 *Districts* are advised to determine a policy on the health care of adolescents, including hospitalisation, which also takes account of the needs of special groups like

- **disabled** young people
- **chronically ill** young people
- young people with **mental health problems**
- young people with **mental handicap**
- young women and girls in hospital for **confinement or termination of pregnancy.**

4.33 An explicit commitment to **family centred care** is advised which through co-operation with parents and community services

- **minimises the length** and frequency of necessary hospital admissions
- provides for **appropriately trained staff** to supervise their care, eg a consultant paediatrician and a RSCN (or a nurse who has completed the children's branch of Project 2000)
- encourages the use of **nurses of both sexes** in the care of adolescent patients.

4.34 Particular regard should be given to the transitional planning of the health care of **adolescents with disabilities or chronic illness.** Under Sections 5 and 6 of the Disabled Persons Act 1986[37], Education Authorities and Social Service Departments are required to liaise on planning the social care needs of children with permanent and substantial handicap from age 14. Health authority staff will participate in assessments of these children, but it is also necessary to ensure continuity in the supervision of their health care. Usually a consultant paediatrician will have taken the lead in respect of chronically sick children and it is necessary to ensure that a consultant in an appropriate adult specialty, whose identity is known to the family and other agencies, takes on the lead role during this transitional period and thereafter. In most cases the consultant will need to take account of the views of both the patients and their parents in devising a programme of care. The study by Exeter University on "The Needs of Handicapped Young Adults"[38] highlights many of the issues that need to be addressed in planning services for this group.

4.35 *Provider hospitals* are advised to consult with *Districts* about meeting their policy requirements. Wherever practical they are advised to provide a separate adolescent unit within the children's department. Where this is impractical, a separate area should be designated within the paediatric unit and a separate care regime devised which will provide the **freedoms and independence** necessary to meet the needs and expectations of adolescent patients.

4.36 Experience suggests that the following facilities are necessary

- space for **privacy** in washing and toilet areas with equipment for disposal of sanitary towels, hairwashing, shaving etc
- space for the use, display and storage of **personal belongings**
- space for education, study and socialising which must be accessible and usable by all categories of patient – youth clubs have been successful at some hospitals
- kitchen facilities which, by allowing patients to make snacks and drinks, give them some **flexibility in the organisation of their day**
- use of a **telephone**
- accommodation for members of the patients' families to stay **overnight.**

4.37 Adolescents need the freedom to wear and care for their own clothes. They rely heavily on contacts with their peer group and visiting from friends should be encouraged as well as from members of the family. They need to be aware of the freedoms and restrictions on matters like use of recreational facilities, leaving ward areas and access for visitors. To meet these needs, *provider hospitals* are advised to issue adolescent patients with written information on **"house rules"** on or before admission to hospital.

Life-Threatening Illness 4.38 Because the incidence of life threatening illnesses and death in childhood is no longer common, health care staff may not have the experience of supporting a family in such circumstances. Recent developments, often initiated by voluntary organisations, have led to a growing consensus on good practice and this is now an area of **very fruitful co-operation** between voluntary organisations, health and local authorities and academic departments. Current good practice reflects medical advances like the improved outcomes, which are being achieved in the treatment of leukaemia and other cancers, and the longer fuller lives which children with some congenital or genetic degenerative diseases are able to live. Parents/carers particularly need **advice and support both on first being informed of the nature of their child's illness and when the options for the child's care are discussed.**

4.39 There is a growing consensus that care should be family centred and flexible in its response to the different needs and circumstances of children and their families. The main preconditions for this model of care are

- **community support** services to help families care for children in their homes
- the availabílity of high quality **respite care** to give families the confidence to take a break from caring for a child at home.

4.40 The book published by Action for the Care of Families whose Children have Life Threatening and Terminal Conditions (ACT) "Listen. My Child has a lot of Living to Do"[39] and the booklet "Care of Dying Children and their Families"[40] are useful reference documents. ACT is also developing a database of voluntary organisations working in this area from which they would be willing to supply information to *districts* and *provider hospitals*. Other organisations such as the Cancer Relief MacMillan Fund contribute to the training and funding of nurses in the care of children with cancer.

4.41 *Districts* and *provider hospitals* are encouraged to establish links with voluntary organisations active in their areas to achieve the maximum degree of co-operation in the planning and organisation of services like domiciliary nursing, social work support and respite care (see paragraphs 5.13-5.16). In agreeing contractual specifications they are advised to ensure that

- all staff working in children's departments (including staff from other agencies such as teachers and social workers) are **sensitive to the needs** of children (and their families) with life-threatening conditions and are able to draw upon staff specifically trained in care and counselling
- parents are informed in an appropriate manner, as soon as possible of their child's condition and given every opportunity to **talk through their feelings**
- **privacy** is available to child and parents
- parents can **participate** actively in the care of their child, along with staff familiar to them to provide support and advice
- children have the opportunity to lead **as full a life** as possible including the opportunity to play
- care is taken at all times not to '**avoid**' parents whose child is dying, while at the same time recognising the need for privacy
- parents can take their child **home to die**, if that is their wish and it is compatible with the medical and nursing care needed
- where children are taken home, there is proper liaison with community and primary care services and advice is available to parents on the help available from statutory or voluntary agencies, to ensure ongoing **support and counselling** for as long as necessary
- throughout the care and treatment of these children full account is taken of any need for the **effective control of pain**
- parents have the opportunity to return to the hospital **to find out anything further they wish to know** about any aspect of their child's illness, care and treatment.

Death of a Child

4.42 When a child dies, it is essential that parents/carers are **helped to cope** with the sense of loss and grief and also given practical assistance to help them make the decisions which the events following death require. *Districts* and *provider hospitals* are advised to ensure that

- in the case of unexpected or sudden bereavement – eg 'accident and emergency' deaths and Sudden Infant Death – parents are able **to wait in a private room** and, if they have to identify the body, that they are given advice beforehand and support during and after the identification
- account is taken of **parents wishes on the observance of death** – including the "laying-out" of their children – this may involve the clothes to be worn, the taking of a photograph or lock of hair for the parents to keep or a brief ceremony
- parents are given the privacy to **grieve alone** in a quiet room set aside for this purpose, with the body of their child (if they so wish) and access to the mortuary to view the child's body
- a member of staff trained in **care and counselling** is designated to give families, including siblings, all the necessary support including help with the arrangement of bereavement counselling and practical issues like burial arrangements
- the results of any post mortem investigation are conveyed in a sympathetic manner to the family – eg in person rather than by telephone – in order that the **therapeutic value** of the discussion of the pathologist's findings is fully realised
- the family's GP is informed as soon as possible in the event of the death of a child so that, as necessary, **the GP can help them cope with the medical effects of bereavement.**

Arrangements for Burial and Cremation

4.43 Hospitals have **a special role** in relation to the burial and cremation of children including stillborn children and children who die shortly after birth. *Districts* and *provider hospitals* are advised to ensure that, in the case of stillbirths and neonatal deaths, the **procedures and arrangements for burial or cremation** are known to staff, and written information is available for the parents which indicates that

- the hospital has an obligation to offer to arrange and **pay for the funeral** of stillborn children (in hospital or community)
- there are arrangements the hospital can make if parents find the funeral costs **beyond their means**
- practical assistance can be provided in transferring babies to the parents' home area if they were stillborn or died in a hospital **outside that area**

4.44 *Provider hospitals* are also advised to ensure that

- a member of staff, familiar with local arrangements, is designated as a **central point of contact** to whom parents can turn, in the first instance, for help and advice
- where a **stillborn or neonatal death support group** exists locally or within the region, bereavement procedures include reference to it (the publication "Miscarriage, Stillbirth and Neonatal death: Guidelines for Professionals" by the Stillbirth and Neonatal Death Society[41] contains relevant good practice)
- hospital arrangements for the burial or cremation of a stillborn baby or a

baby who dies shortly after birth are **dignified**, involving a simple ceremony if the parents wish

- hospital staff have a knowledge of the **religious customs and observances** relating to death in Christian and non- Christian faiths
- the site of burial is a specially designated, well-kept area
- **parents' wishes** for any observance on death are accommodated – **eg a brief ceremony**
- that the hospital can assist with taking a **photograph** of the child for the parents to keep.

The Protection of Children from Abuse

4.45 Hospital staff in contact with children need to be alert to indications of child abuse. The DHSS guide "Working Together"[42] notes that **abused children may attend hospital accident and emergency departments** as a consequence of injuries inflicted upon them and that staff working in these departments may need to seek specialist advice – eg from a consultant paediatrician – to assess whether there are signs of a history of abuse. Staff in children's departments will also have major contributions to make to the continuing care of abused children and may have a formal role in the legislative and procedural framework for the investigation and prevention of child abuse.

4.46 Social Service Departments have the primary responsibility for the protection of children, but need the co-operation of other agencies in planning and providing services. SSD's should take the lead in establishing **Area Child Protection Committees (ACPCs),** the inter-agency committees for developing, monitoring and reviewing child protection policies. Working Together [42] recommends that ACPCs include representatives of health service management, medical and psychiatric services and nursing services. The SSD is responsible for providing the secretariat and support services for the committee and normally for providing the Chairman. The guide also suggests that **Special Assessment Teams (SATS)** – comprising a social worker, a doctor and a police officer – be formed where a multi-disciplinary assessment is considered necessary to determine, in a case of suspected sexual abuse, whether there is cause for concern which requires further investigation or other action.

4.47 *Districts* and *provider units* should ensure that

- hospital staff working with children are **trained to recognise** the symptoms of child abuse and are aware of how they can obtain specialist expert advice and support
- there are sound procedures for **acting upon suspicion of child abuse** which cover the role of other agencies – eg SSDs and police
- there is **provision in contracts** for specialist medical nursing staff to participate in multi-agency forums for the prevention of child abuse – eg ACPC's, SATs.

4.48 It is for the SSD to provide a **Place of Safety** for children at risk of abuse unless treatment or medical or nursing assessment is necessary. Where there are clinical reasons for the admission of a child to hospital it should still be possible for the SSD to designate a hospital ward as a place of safety, a principle which will also apply from October 1991 following implementation of Section 44 of the Children Act[43], under a Care and Protection Order. Otherwise it will be inappropriate for children at risk of abuse to be admitted to a children's ward as a place of safety unless there is a clinical reason to support this action.

Security

4.49 The benefits to the child of being accompanied by a parent/carer while in hospital **fully justify the additional measures** a hospital needs to take to ensure that their access to a children's ward does not pose a threat to security. Nevertheless, *Districts* and *provider hospitals* are advised to ensure that

- the unrestricted access of parents and other visitors to children's wards **does not jeopardise the children's safety**
- doors of wards, which will normally be unlocked during the day to allow free movement of staff and visitors, **are secured at night**, whether or not parents are staying with their children (The Department of Health Fire Code[44] provides advice on the fire safety aspects of security in hospital including the use of locks which permit exit without the use of a key)
- staff caring for the children are alert to the presence of strangers by their knowlege of who are legitimate visitors (if their credentials are checked, the presence of parents on the ward may act as an added deterrent to any would-be intruder).

4.50 Further guidance on security issues can be found in the **NHS Security Manual**, published by the National Association of Health Authorities and Trusts[45]. An updated version should be available in late 1991.

Children and Diet

4.51 **Good feeding** is essential to the welfare of children in hospital and can play a vital part in their recovery from treatment. Food provides a continuing link with the home, it is often associated with treats and rewards and its consumption should induce a feeling of well being. When considering the catering requirements of children, *provider hospitals* are advised to take the following information into account

- **current nutritional advice**
- the needs of children of differing age groups, in relation to the **size, content and timing of meals**
- the provision of a **choice** of meals that children will like
- any **special dietary considerations** (see paragraphs 4.25-4.27 on children from ethnic minority backgrounds)
- the provision of **cutlery and utensils** suitable for children of different ages and any feeding aids required by children with special needs.

4.52 If it is found that a child is not eating an adequate diet from the hospital menu, parents can be invited to bring in more familiar food, provided there is no contra-indication and that the food is not given to other children. The expert advice of a dietitian may be called upon if necessary.

Oral Health Care

4.53 *Provider hospitals* are advised that all children in hospital require **daily mouth care** supervised, and assisted where necessary by nursing staff. An emergency dental service should be available for children who are admitted for short-stays. Comprehensive dental services need to be provided to longer-stay patients under the supervision of a consultant in paediatric dentistry.

5: Other locally provided Services for Children

Comprehensive Assessment

5.1 In addition to the need for assessments arising out of child health surveillance, there are the following **statutory requirements** for the assessment of children's needs and abilities over the age range 0-19

- assessment of **special educational needs** under the Education Act 1981[28]
- assessment of **disability** under the Chronically Sick and Disabled Persons Act 1970[46] and the Disabled Persons Act 1986[37]
- assessment of **need** under section 17 of the Children Act 1989[43]
- assessments undertaken in accordance with a Child Assessment Order made under section 43 of the Children Act 1989[43] when it is **suspected that a child is suffering or is likely to suffer significant harm**

5.2 Collaboration between the different authorities with lead responsibility for these functions is encouraged to ensure that the needs of the child and family are assessed **"in the round"**. The Children Act[43] provides for the assessment of a child's needs to be made at the same time as that made under any other enactment. In all assessments it is essential that due account is taken of the child's health and development, any disabilities, educational needs including **special educational needs, religion, racial origin, cultural and linguistic background**, together with the family circumstances and parents'/carers knowledge and understanding of their own child.

5.3 *Districts* should agree policies on the arrangement of child assessment and collaborative working arrangements with Social Service Departments and Local Education Authorities. In deciding how a health care contribution to assessment can be secured, *Districts* should be aware that the use of **Child Development Teams** (sometimes referred to as District Handicap Teams) has proved successful in many districts. The core membership of these teams usually comprises

- the **consultant paediatrician** (community child health)
- a **paediatric nurse** with specific experience of children with disabilities
- a **specialist social worker**
- a clinical or educational **psychologist**
- a **teacher** experienced in teaching children with special educational needs

5.4 The team will also need to have available to it appropriate clinical specialists from all the **relevant disciplines** and there should be good liaison arrangements with the child's GP and health visitor. The contribution of speech therapists, physiotherapists, occupational therapists and play specialists should be clearly recognised and incorporated. Usually, but not necessarily, the consultant paediatrician leads the team. It is important that the **family be involved** in all aspects of the child's assessment.

5.5 Increasingly, assessments are being carried out in the community, but where a *District* and its *provider units* agree an assessment unit should be located in a hospital, they are advised to consider provision of the following facilities

- **a consulting room** for examinations and assessment
- **a play room**
- a suitably equipped room for **ophthalmology**
- a sound-proofed room for **audiology and speech therapy**
- space for **physiotherapy**
- **specialised facilities** for assessment and treatment (eg playroom with one-way mirror)
- facilities for **occupational therapy**
- facilities to aid **rehabilitation** eg wheelchairs and orthoses
- facilities for **office staff**, records and equipment
- **waiting space** for parents and children (including private space for changing and feeding babies and children, play space, and a secure area for leaving prams, push-chairs etc).

5.6 Adequate accommodation, able to be used **flexibly,** should be provided within the paediatric unit for all disciplines involved in the multi- disciplinary assessment of children with special needs and a wide range of disabling conditions.

Children with mental handicap

5.7 The organisation of care for children with mental handicap has undergone a major transformation in recent years. As noted in "Caring for People"[47], the objective since 1981 that no child requiring long-term residential care should grow up in a large mental handicap hospital has been very largely achieved. The changes proposed in "Caring for People" mean that when the new local authority forms of service are sufficiently developed, children with a mental handicap should, like other children, only be in hospital when they have medical **or nursing needs which cannot be met otherwise by primary or community health services.**

5.8 However, the need for local authorities and health authorities to **work together** to ensure that the health and developmental needs of children with mental handicap are met remains of paramount importance. When general hospital services are required, the children should attend or be admitted to the paediatric department. In placing contracts for hospital services *districts* are advised to ensure that for children with a mental handicap

- arrangements exist for **good communication** between the hospital and the child's usual carer, general practitioner, community health staff and school
- consideration is given to the role of **hospital** paediatric staff (eg consultant paediatrician, clinical psychologist, play specialists, nurses, physiotherapists, occupational and speech therapists) in the regular monitoring and assessment of the health and development of children with mental handicap **outside** the hospital.

5.9 **Respite care** provides essential support to families caring for children with mental handicap (see paragraphs 5.13-5.16)

5.10 The Department is to issue guidance on the care of children with disabilities including mental handicap in the series of guidance on implementation of the Children Act 1989[45]

Child and Adolescent Psychiatry

5.11 The cardinal principles in part 2 of this guide apply to children and young people whenever they are admitted to hospital. Children and adolescents who develop **serious mental health problems** – eg anorexia – requiring in-patient hospital care should be treated in specialist hospital units. Good liaison should be established between staff working in general paediatric departments and the child and adult mental health services so that **expertise, guidance and advice may be shared** to the benefit of the children and their families.

5.12 *Districts* are advised to consider their needs for **specialist hospital child psychiatry and psychology services** when contracting for children's hospital services. Good practices on services for disturbed young people and adolescents were the subject of the Health Advisory Service report "Bridge Over Troubled Waters"[48]. In respect of general hospital services, *district* and *provider* hospitals are advised to agree that specialist mental health care staff are available to the children's department for advice when

- children are failing to thrive and **psychological factors** are suspected of contributing to their condition
- a child or family's reaction to the illness is **impeding the child's recovery**
- the nature of a child's condition is such that he/she is likely to be **severely distressed** – eg in cases of prolonged immobility from an orthopaedic condition, life-threatening or terminal illnesses, unpleasant treatments such as bone marrow transplantation, chemotherapy, radiotherapy, skin grafts and amputations
- a child is felt to be at **risk of mental, physical, or sexual abuse**
- a child has carried out an act of **deliberate self-harm**.

Respite Care

5.13 The availability of **accessible, good quality respite care** is essential for the delivery of a high standard of family centred child health care in which one of the primary roles of the health services and other agencies should be to support families to care for their children in the home.

5.14 Respite care can help families caring for children with

- **chronic illness or disability**
- **life threatening illness**
- **mental handicap or mental illness.**

5.15 The aim should be to provide a safe, stimulating environment in which parents/carers feel confident in leaving their children for short stays. As far as practicable the children need a continuation of the care regime to which they have been accustomed at home in facilities located in the local community. A **hospital children's department is not an appropriate place for the provision of respite care**, unless the child concerned has specific health care needs which can only be safely met in a hospital environment. Usually the treatment needs of children cared for at home can be met by parents/carers with the support provided by community health staff like paediatric community nurses. In such circumstances the primary need is for social care without the restrictions which an acute hospital environment inevitably puts on everyday living. Some local authorities have specialist family based fostering placements which are supported by primary and community health staff.

5.16 *Districts* are advised to assess the respite care needs of children within their resident populations and, in collaboration with Social Service Departments and appropriate voluntary organisations, agree plans for meeting these needs. In some areas voluntary organisations have developed high quality facilities available for the use of families with children who have life threatening or terminal conditions (see paragraphs 4.38 - 4.41). Since these are sometimes children with quite complex medical needs who might otherwise have to be cared for in hospital, it seems appropriate for *Districts* to contract for services with such organisations – **subject to the regular monitoring of the quality of the service provided**. For other children the SSD may be better placed to make the most appropriate arrangements. The use of community hospitals distant from the DGH to provide respite care is unlikely to be appropriate, even for children requiring a high level of health care support, unless it is possible to make discrete provision for children's care in line with the general principles of this guide.

Chaplaincy

5.17 It is recognised that children develop spiritual awareness from a very early age. Hospital staff need to be sensitive to children's needs and wishes for spiritual support. Adolescents may likewise have their own individual need of religious guidance. Many families feel the need for spiritual support and comfort when children are ill, particularly when a chronic or life threatening illness is diagnosed. Hospital chaplains make a vital contribution both to the care of children and young people in hospital and to the support of their families.

5.18 *Districts* and *Provider hospitals* are advised to ensure

- that the **services of the chaplain are available** to children and their families
- **chaplains are fully involved** in relevant training programmes (for example, in the care of distressing conditions and bereavement counselling) whether in a teaching or learning capacity or simply by sharing experiences with other staff involved in the care of children.

5.19 Where ecumenical and inter-faith practices are encouraged in the community, the hospital chaplain, who is generally from the Church of England, can be very supportive to families whatever their religious affiliation. This should not detract from the right of any family to be visited by their own parish priest or minister if they so wish. Staff will also wish to bear in mind the spiritual needs of families from non-Christian faiths, and ensure access to their religious advisers as appropriate (see also paragraph 4.25).

6: Staffing and Training

In agreeing staffing specifications in their contracts for children's services, *Districts* and *provider hospitals* should be guided by the following principles.

Medical Staff

6.1 Every child admitted to a hospital children's department should be supervised by a **children's physician or surgeon**. Where, exceptionally, a child is admitted to another department, a named paediatric consultant should be responsible for advising the consultant concerned on the care and treatment of this child. In addition

- a consultant paediatrician should be responsible for giving advice on care and treatment policies in maternity and accident and emergency units and a senior paediatrician should be available 24 hours a day to give **cover** to these departments
- staff rosters should provide for adequate **safety net cover** in both the children's department and the other departments where paediatric support is required
- facilities should be available, with appropriate protected time, for the **training of paediatric staff** in accordance with the requirements of the Royal College of Physicians. At consultant level, time and facilities will need to be provided for medical audit and postgraduate training
- in other specialties regularly involved in the care of children – eg anaesthetics, general surgery, ENT, opthalmology, radiology and pathology – there should be consultants, **trained and experienced** in the treatment of children, available to participate in and advise on their treatment†.
- the District General Hospital will normally accommodate the child psychiatric department, which should have a close relationship with the children's department, to ensure that both the **physical and emotional needs** of all the children receiving hospital care are met – joint rounds by paediatricians and child psychiatrists and joint out-patient clinics are examples of how this relationship has developed.

† The Report of the National Confidential Enquiry into Perioperative Deaths 1989[49] found that the outcome of surgery and anaesthesia in children is related to the experience of the clinicians involved and recommended that surgeons and anaesthetists should not undertake occasional paediatric practice.

Nursing Staff

6.2 It is accepted that the general nursing needs of children can best be met by grouping them in a discrete children's department with an experienced RSCN in charge **supported by other nurses qualified in the care of children**. The introduction of day care, day wards and the extension in the range of out-patient treatments and paediatric community nursing services has resulted in those children admitted to hospital being more acutely ill than in the past with higher dependency and considerably increased throughput. This, together with the related need to educate and support families so they are competent to care for their children, has accentuated the need for registered paediatric trained nursing staff in children's departments.

6.3 In agreeing contractual specifications for the nurse staffing of children's hospital services, *Districts* and *provider hospitals* are advised to take account of the following standards

- there are *at least two* Registered Sick Children's Nurses (RSCN) (or nurses who have completed the child branch of Project 2000) on duty **24 hours a day** in all hospital children's departments and wards
- there is a RSCN available 24 hours a day to advise on the **nursing of children in other departments** – eg the intensive care unit, the A&E department, out-patients
- there should be sufficient RSCNs to **supervise the training of student nurses** (from 1995 it will be a requirement of the English National Board for Nursing, Midwifery and Health Visiting that nurse students on children's wards are supervised by a RSCN at all times)
- the RSCN/child ratio staff numbers and skill mix should be commensurate with patient needs and **determined by a systematic method of manpower demand assessment** which is regularly reviewed – guidance is available in Dear Administrator letter DA(87) 12 on Nurse Manpower Planning[50].

Nursery Nurses

6.4 Nursery nurses undertake a two year training course in the care of well children 0-7 years and they can make a very valuable contribution to the physical and emotional needs of children in children's wards and other hospital departments – eg in bathing, dressing and feeding sick and convalescent children, and acting as substitute parents where they are unable to be present. *Districts* and *provider hospitals* should ensure this contribution **never extends to duties appropriate to a registered or enrolled nurse**. The ENB letter to Regional Nursing Officers "The Role and Responsibilities of Nursery Nurses in Paediatric Units, Including Special Care Baby Units"[51] refers.

Health Care Assistants

6.5 The training of health care assistants is still under development, but, as with nursery nurses, their use on children's wards **should be supervised by a nurse qualified in the care of children.**

Other Staff

6.6 There is a **wide range of professionals** who have an important contribution to make to the care and treatment of children and should be available to work in the children's department eg clinical psychologists, speech therapists, audiologists, physiotherapists, occupational therapists, dietitians, play specialists, clerical and ancillary staff and, staff from other agencies such as teachers. They all need training and experience in the care of sick children, child development and communicating sympathetically with parents/carers and other family members.

6.7 **Social workers** also have an essential contribution to make to the welfare of children and their families and there need to be collaborative arrangements with Social Service Departments to ensure that they receive training appropriate in child health care.

6.8 Professional and technical staff in X-ray departments, laboratories, pharmacies and other support services will require **training in the special demands** that the treatment of children make upon these services – eg the micro-method investigation which should form the basis of much of the work in children's pathology.

Training

6.9 The education and training implications of the NHS Review for non-medical staff were first considered in Working Paper 10 in the Working for Patients series[52] and developed in subsequent Executive Letters. Under the new arrangements:

- *Regional Health Authorities* will play a key role by assessing **demand** for training, and allocating funds to ensure its supply
- *Districts* as purchasers of services will have **no direct role** in assessing levels of demand for training, although the adequacy of trained staff is likely to be a factor they consider when awarding contracts
- *Provider units* will be responsible for **determining their staffing needs** and planning and managing the training and career development of the staff required to meet them.

6.10 The main principles of guidance on funding issues given in EL(90)171[53] are

- in the longer term *Regions* will be expected to fund all of their training needs from their general allocations
- for an initial period **a pragmatic approach** will need to be adopted to distinguish between the value of the service contribution provided to units by staff under training from the training costs they incur.

6.11 The implications for the main staff groups involved in children's care are as follows

- for **pre-registration nurse training** (RGN, RMN, RSCN, EN and equivalent Project 2000 courses), costs of running courses will be met by the English National Board and RHAs while salaries will be paid by the employing units who will reclaim the training elements from RHAs
- for **post-registration training** for nurses such as the ENB course in Paediatric Intensive Care, RHAs will be identifying current investment by health authorities in recordable and other post-registration courses in terms of post-registration tutor salaries and associated costs (but not including trainees salaries) to form the baseline for a budget for the 1991/92 financial year
- for **physiotherapy** training, RHAs will have the sole responsibility for bursaries and the cost of running courses
- for **speech therapy** training, at present the only cost borne by the NHS is that of clinical placements, which is offset to a limited extent by the

contribution students make to patient care – (these arrangements are being reviewed and guidance on funding and the costing of clinical placements issued)

- for **hearing therapists**, training is currently centrally organised but locally funded (discussions are currently underway about future arrangements)
- for **occupational therapy**, the central training budget held by the Department will be allocated to RHAs with effect from September 1991, from when RHAs will make arrangements to pay bursaries and course costs
- most candidates for **play specialist** training are already employed by *provider units* who bear the cost of release. RHAs will become responsible for the cost of course and examination fees the guidance on the costing of clinical placement will be relevant to the assessment of the costs of day release.

Sources of Guidance on Staff Requirements and Training

6.12 It is for *provider hospitals* to determine the numbers of these staff they will require to meet their contractual obligations. Guidance is available from the following sources

- for medical staff, from the **British Paediatric Association**
- for nursing staff, including RSCNs and nurses in Intensive Care Units, from the **English National Board for Nursing Midwifery and Health Visiting**
- for speech therapists from the **College of Speech Therapists**
- for hospital play specialists from the **National Association of Hospital Play Staff Specialists**
- for teachers and non-teaching assistants from **Local Education Authorities**
- for other staff, from the **relevant professional association**

7: Conclusion

Advances in medical science, changes in the delivery of health care and perhaps a better understanding of children's developmental needs will all lead to further innovation and refinement. The guidance we are to prepare on community child health services will examine in closer detail the relationship between hospital and community services in areas like hospital discharge, day care and the care of children with disabilities. Nevertheless we feel that there are very few districts in which use of this guide would not improve the quality of children's health care.

Throughout preparation of the guidance we have been conscious of the commitment and dedication shown to children in the health services – by NHS staff, staff of other state agencies concerned with children, members of professional bodies and staff associations and the legion of voluntary workers who give so much both individually and as members of voluntary organisations. Because of this commitment we know that the guidance will be subject to critical evaluation and we would welcome feedback on its use and further development. Comments or suggestions should be sent to the Department's Child Health Section (CMP1C) in Wellington House, 133 – 155 Waterloo Road, London, SE1 8UG.

Appendix A

References

1 *The Welfare of Children in Hospital – Report of the Platt Committee.* Published in 1959. Available from HMSO bookshops.

2 *Fit for the Future – Report of the Court Committee on Child Health Services.* Available from HMSO.

3 *Working for Patients – Starting Specifications: A DHA Project.* Available from NHS Management Executive, Richmond House, 79 Whitehall, London SW1A 2NS.

4 *The NAWCH Quality Review – Setting Standards for children in Health Care.* Available from NAWCH Ltd. Argyle House, 29/31 Euston Road, London NW1 2SD

5 *Circular HC(91)2 – Medical Audit in the Hospital and Community Health Services.* *

6 *NAWCH Charter.* Available from NAWCH Ltd address as at 4.

7 *Overview of Research on the Care of Children in Hospital.* Published by the University of Warwick. Available from the Department of Sociology University of Warwick, Coventry CV4 7AL.

8 *Guide to Consent for Examination or Treatment.* Published by NHS Management Executive. Address as at 3.

9 *Research Involving Patients.* Published by the Royal College of Physicians, 11 St. Andrews Place, London NW1.

10 *Nursing Children in the Accident and Emergency Department.* Available from the Royal College of Nursing, 20 Cavendish Square, London W1M 30B.

11 *Circular HN(84)25/LASS(84)5 – Health Services Management: The Management of Deliberate Self Harm.* *

12 *Circular HC(89)5 – Discharge of Patients from Hospitals.* *

13 *Hidden Children – an analysis of ward attenders in children's wards.* Published by Caring for Children in the Health Services, 7 Belgrave Place, Clifton, Bristol, BS8 3DD.

14 *Just for the Day – Children admitted to Hospital for Day Treatment.* Available from CCHS address as at 13.

15 *Organisation and Costs of Day Surgery.* Published by the NHS Management Executive Value for Money Unit. Available from NHSME Value for Money Unit, 286 Euston Road, London NW1 3DN.

16 *The Maternity Services Advisory Committee (MSAC) 3rd Report.* Available from Department of Health, PO Box 21, Stanmore, Middlesex, HA7 1DY.

17 *British Paediatric Association Working Party Report on Paediatric Intensive Care.* Available from British Paediatric Association, 5 St. Andrews Place, Regents Park, London NW1 4LB.

18 *Hospital Building Note No. 23 – Hospital Accommodation for Children.* *

19 *CMO Letter PL/CMO(89)4 – HIV Infection, Breastfeeding and Human Milk Banking in the United Kingdom.* *

20 *Parents Staying Overnight with their Children.* Available from CCHS address as at 13.

21 *Leaflet H11 – NHS Travel Costs Scheme.* *

22 *Quality Management for Children: Play in Hospital.* Available from Save the Children Fund, UK Department, 17 Grove Lane, London SE5 8RD.

23 *Hospital: A Deprived Environment for Children ? The Case for Hospital Playschemes.* Available from Save the Children Fund address as at 22.

24 *Department of Education & Science Circular 5/89.* Available from DES Publication Dispatch Centre, Honeypot Lane, Stanmore, Middlesex, HA7 1DY.

25 *HMI Report – Hospital and Home Tuition.* Available from DES address as at 24.

26 *Hospital and Home Education Services.* Available from DES address as at 24.

27 *Education Act 1944.* Available from HMSO.

28 *Education Act 1981.* Available from HMSO.

29 *Department of Education & Science Design Note 38.* Available from DES address as at 24.

30 *Circular HSC(IS)37 – The Education of Mentally Handicapped Young Children in Hospital.* *

31 *Circular HN(89)20 – Assessments and Statements of Special Educational Needs: Procedures within the Education, Health and Social Services.* *

32 *Action Not Words – A Strategy to Improve Health Services for Black and Ethnic Minority Groups.* Available from NAHAT, Birmingham Research Park, Vincent Drive, Birmingham, B15 2SQ.

33 *Health Care in Multiracial Britain.* Published by the Health Education Authority/National Extension College. Available from HEA, Hamilton House, Mabledon Street, London WC1X 9TX.

34 *Traveller Mothers and Babies.* Available from The Maternity Alliance, 15 Britannia Street, London, WC1X 9JP.

35 *Setting Standards for Children and Adolescents in Hospital.* Available from NAWCH address as at 4.

36 *British Paediatric Association Working Party Report on the Needs and Care of Adolescents (1985).* Available from BPA address as at 17.

37 *Disabled Persons (Services Consultation And Representation) Act 1986.* Available from HMSO.

38 *The Needs of Handicapped Young Children.* Published by Exeter University. Available from Exeter University, Publications Office, Reed Mews, Streatham Drive, Exeter, Devon.

39 *Listen. My Child has a lot of Living to do.* Published by Oxford University Press, in association with the Institute of Child Health Bristol.

40 *The Care of Dying Children and their Families.* Available from NAHAT address as at 32.

41 *Miscarriage, Stillbirth and Neonatal Death: Guidelines for Professionals.* Available from the Stillbirth and Neonatal Death Society 28 Portland Place, London W1N 4DF.

42 *Working Together – A guide to arrangements for inter-agency co-operation for the protection of children from abuse.* Available from HMSO. To be revised during 1991.

43 *Children Act 1989.* Available from HMSO.

44 *Department of Health Fire Code.* Available from HMSO.

45 *NHS Security Manual.* Available from NAHAT address as at 32.

46 *Chronically Sick and Disabled Persons Act 1970.* Available from HMSO.

47 *Caring for People.* Published by the Department of Health. Available from HMSO.

48 *Bridge Over Troubled Waters.* Published by NHS Advisory Service. Available from HMSO.

49 *The Report of the National Confidential Enquiry into Perioperative Deaths (1989).* Available from HMSO.

50 *Dear Administrator Letter DA(87)12 Nurse Manpower Planning.* *

51 *English Nursing Board Letter – The Role and Responsibilities of Nursery Nurses in Paediatric Units, including Special Care Baby Units.* Available from English Nursing Board, Victory House, 170 Tottenham Court Road, London W1P 0HA.

52 *Working Paper 10 in Working for Patients series.* Available from HMSO.

53 *Executive Letter EL(90)171 – Non-Medical Education and Training: Guidance on Funding Issues* *

*   Available from Department of Health, Health Publications Unit, No.2 Site, Manchester Road, Heywood, Lancs. OL10 2PZ.

Appendix B

Bibliography

Health for All Children – A Programme for Child Health Surveillance. Edited by David M B Hall. Oxford Medical Publications 1989.

Child Abuse And Neglect: Facing the Challenge. Editors Wendy Stainton Rogers, Denise Hevey and Elizabeth Ash. Oxford University Press

An Introduction to The Children Act 1989. HMSO

Immunisation Against Infectious Disease 1990. HMSO

Depression After Child Birth. K Dalton. Published by Oxford University Press

Coping with Young Children. J Douglas. Published by Penguin.

Coping with Your Handicapped Child. A E McCormack. Published by Chambers.

Child Health in a Multicultural Society (2nd edition). John Black. Published by BMJ Publications.

Where are the Children? An Examination of Regional Statistics for Children in Hospital and their Implications Regarding Agreed Standards of Care. Published by Caring for Children in the Health Services.

Guidelines for Day Case Surgery. Published by The Royal College of Surgeons of England.

Joint Statement on Children's Attendances at Accident and Emergency Departments. Published by British Paediatric Association, British Association of Paediatric Surgeons and Casualty Surgeons Association.

Investing in the Future – Child Health Ten Years After The Court Report. Published by National Children's Bureau.

The Integration of Child Health Services: An Introduction. Published by British Paediatric Association.

Promoting Better Health: The Government's Programme for Improving Primary Health Care. HMSO.

Immunisation Against Infectious Diseases. DHSS Joint Committee on Vaccination and Immunisation. HMSO.

Basic Principles of Child Accident Prevention : A Guide to Action. Published by Child Accident Prevention Trust.

The Management Response to Childhood Accidents: A Guide to Effective use of NHS Information. Published by Kings Fund Centre.

Research with Children: Ethics, Law and Practice. Published by Institute of Medical Ethics.

Criteria for Care: The Manual of the North West Nurse Staffing Levels Project. Published by Newcastle upon Tyne Polytechnic Products Ltd.

Guidelines for the Workload of Consultant Paediatricians. Published by British Paediatric Association.

Junior Medical Staffing in Paediatric Units. Published by British Paediatric Association.

The Mechanism for Integrating the Child Health Services: A Policy Statement. Published by British Paediatric Association.

Report of the Child Health Forum (1987) Published by British Medical Association.

Sick Children's Nurses: A Study for the DHSS of the Career Patterns of RSCN's. Published by Institute of Manpower Studies, University of Sussex.

A Policy for Play ? Report of a National Conference. Published by Play in Hospital Liaison Committee.

Sudden Infant Death – Patterns, Puzzles and Problems. Published by Open Books Publishing Ltd.

After Stillbirth and Neonatal Death What Happens Next ?. Published by the Stillbirth and Neonatal Death Society.

Hospital at Home: The Coming Revolution. Published by the King's Fund Centre Communications Unit.

Community Paediatric Nursing in England in 1988. An unpublished report available from the Society of Paediatric Nursing at the Royal College of Nursing.

Child Care and the Growth of Love by John Bowlby. Published by Penguin.

Attachment by John Bowlby. Published by Penguin.

Separation by John Bowlby. Published by Penguin.

Loss: Sadness and Depression by John Bowlby. Published by Penguin.

Medical Research with Children – Ethics, Law and Practice by R H Nicholson. Published by the Oxford University Press.

Choosing for Children: Parents Consent to Surgery by Priscilla Anderson. Published by the Oxford University Press.

Printed in the United Kingdom for HMSO
Dd 293829 C100   6/91   531/3 12521